Tending To Your Garden:
How Ayurveda Can Support
A Thriving Pregnancy

Includes 10 Ayurvedic Practices

A Foundational Guide Book By

Viji Natarajan

Divine Journey, LLC

Divine Journey, LLC

Ordering Information:
For bulk ordering or additional book questions, email info@divinejourney.org

Tending to Your Garden: How Ayurveda Can Support a Thriving Pregnancy / Vijayalakshmi Natarajan. —1st ed.
ISBN 9781736128909

CONTENTS

This book is dedicated to all the women who have allowed me the privilege to be a part of their birth journey. Without them, I would not have been able to witness life's incredible miracles daily.

FOREWORD

One of the greatest hobbies I started in my 40s was gardening. Every day, I am blown away by the miracle of life and am amazed at the intense similarities between taking care of our bodies and taking care of a garden. I also began to see how the approach I try to teach my clients towards pregnancy, labor, and delivery is equally relevant when I wait every day for the seed I planted to break ground! Not only do I have to show patience and compassion towards my garden, but I must also offer it to myself!

Over the past decade, I've witnessed the difference in outcomes when you look at birth as a single moment vs. a part of a continuous journey. When we think of birth as a journey, we understand that we can affect what happens all along the way. It is not only about breathing through a contraction or whether you use pain management. When you holistically prepare for birth, you can even impact the length and pain experience of labor well before you even arrive at the hospital!

My passion for deliberately supporting women through their childbirth journey using Ayurveda comes from wanting every mother to have a healthy, happy, and non-traumatic birth. Ayurveda is a medical science from India and believes that health is not defined through the lens of a singular moment but a totality of our existence. This changes with time and circumstance. If you understand that our existence is connected to nature, you have already aligned yourself with Ayurveda's principles. When you use Ayurvedic principles for your birth journey, it is only natural that you will impact your labor and delivery as you affect your overall wellness.

One of my clients said it well:

> While Viji and I certainly did discuss the practical aspects of the birth and the sequence of events and options that would be presented to me the day of, the true groundwork and progress for how well my

delivery went were made through self-awareness and simple things that at the start of my journey seemed almost entirely unrelated to birth. Because the birth of a child does not exist in isolation, but in the context of my life - my own physical, mental and spiritual well-being, my continual journey of self-growth, my relationships with those I loved – these elements proved to be far more important than the decisions such as what pain medications I intended for the actual day of birth.

In relation to birth, this self-growth manifested into a newfound sense of confidence in myself and the process and ability to be at ease with birth. Even the delivery not happening as I intended (as should be expected with a complex, biological process such as birth) did not interfere with how perfectly it turned out. My birth journey had already prepared me for all one can prepare for and mentally gotten me to a place to gracefully accept the elements you cannot control and embrace the story however it turns out. Through my birth journey, I was able to find a new sense of peace with who I am, strength and trust in my own body, processing my emotions, and improving my relationships.

It is genuinely possible to prepare for and have a non-traumatic birth experience, free of complications. This book will outline simple, straightforward, and accessible Ayurvedic practices to create a supportive physiological and mental environment. It will help you prepare your body for childbirth and empower you to build strong relationships with your loved ones. Incorporating Ayurvedic practices into your daily routine will promote positive mental, physical, and spiritual well-being and prepare your body for a smoother, less painful, and faster birth than traditional methods. Giving birth doesn't have to be a harrowing experience. With my guidance, you can bring your child into the world free of burden, with excitement, optimism, and energy, all while strengthening your relationship with your partner and yourself.

CHAPTER ONE

A Mother's Story

"Birth is an opportunity to transcend. To rise above what we are accustomed to, reach deeper inside ourselves than we are familiar with, and to see not only what we are truly made of, but the strength we can access in and through birth."

- Marcie Macari

Through my private Ayurvedic Women's Reproductive health practice, I've had the privilege of helping thousands of women through their birth journey. We've managed to avoid cesareans and achieve greater than 98% vaginal births, shorter and faster deliveries with minimal tearing. I attribute such great results to incorporating Ayurveda as the foundational practice and guidance in their pregnancy. Oversight into all aspects that influence a person's journey honors the wholeness of the human experience. It also allows for more profound, long-lasting healing to create health and good outcomes.

Elaine is a client who experienced a joyous and calm labor, complication-free birth, zero perineal tearing, and a healthy baby. Before her delivery, the breakthrough she had with connecting her mind and body allowed her to have the birth she could not even have imagined! This story and hundreds of stories like it fill me with zeal to wake up every day to dedicate my life to sharing the practice of Ayurveda with all mothers and mothers to be.

Elaine's story:

> As a new mom to three-month-old baby girl Genevieve, I am writing my birth story in a place all too familiar to most parents. It is 1 AM, and I sit in a darkened room, dimly lit with the glow of the computer screen, filled with the whirl of a white noise maker. Next to me is my sleeping baby, the other main character in this transitional birth moment. While I hope this story will encourage all women, it is to you, my daughter, that I want to tell this story to most.

> Becoming a mom is the most extraordinary ordinary thing. The ability to support and grow life is a precious gift that comes with great responsibility. It is a universal experience that bonds all mothers, where elements of every mother's story resonate. We have all experienced the immense joy of our baby's first fluttery kicks in our bellies that also comes along with

uncertainty, the fear of whether we will be good mothers.

When I always imagined becoming a mom, I hoped to be at my best. To be a role model in taking care of my body, to be mentally prepared and be grounded. To know where I am going and have accomplished great things so that I could focus solely on you when you arrived. I always thought life was divided into two separate parts – life before becoming a mother and life after. And life after, as I thought, I am the best, evolved, and final version of myself so that I can devote all my energy to you, rather than to myself.

Thus, needless to say, when I learned I was pregnant with you, I was a mixed bag of emotions. These questions subconsciously plagued me – how can I be a good mother if I am still a work in progress myself. How will it be possible to accomplish the things I haven't done yet when I have a whole other human for whom I am responsible? How can I look forward to becoming a mom if the rite of passage is suffering through pregnancy and birth? It seemed raising a child was a combination of exuberant joy attenuated by excruciating pain. Becoming pregnant only made me less sure of myself – as I now had to reconcile my new identity as a mom and the sacrifices that come with it with who I am as an individual.

And to be honest, I was deathly afraid of birth. And why shouldn't I have been? Every exposure I had involved a recounting of the trauma and pain endured by a new mom. My medical school classes certainly didn't help either, as everyone recoiled in horror when we learned about episiotomies to prevent fourth-degree perineal tears that would involve a lifetime of urinary and fecal incontinence. My mother labored for 18+ hours, and the swollen face in my newborn photo gave away the forceps that barely saved her from an emergent C-section. I had no idea how I would get through it, and this fear made me uncertain if I ever even wanted to try.

After five months of pregnancy, I still had no idea and, on some level, just accepted, as many women do, that this would be something I would have to endure somehow. Through a series of fortunate events, I read the birth story of a colleague I had met randomly in passing at an interview. She shared with me the Ayurvedic practitioner to whom she attributed the success of her birth. Viji specialized in women's health - specifically birth - and had somehow excellent testimonials of mom after mom who had experienced fantastic births. I was intrigued, if not cautious about being overly optimistic.

Your dad convinced me to work with her because, after all, this would probably be the most physically and mentally demanding event I would have to go through. If there was anything that we felt worthwhile to spend money on, it was life experiences. We decided it would be valuable if there were even a chance to turn one of the most dreaded days into a more positive one. And in turn, we were told that the domino effect of this positivity would not only permeate the event of birth itself but all things tied to it, both past, present, and future.

As we started our work together, I diligently followed the dietary recommendations based on my constitution and imbalance, as nausea and digestion problems were the predominant symptoms plaguing me the past five months. While I did feel much better, I still had off days, and those off days would lead to me veering off course, which would lead to more nausea and indigestion, and the cycle would start all over again. Through this, I gained awareness of what my body needed, but feeling unwell made it hard to follow every day—feeling ill permeated beyond just my digestion but also into every other aspect of my life. I lacked the motivation to take care of my body and struggled to get through my workday with my low energy levels. I had a poor attitude towards my loved ones and, thus, also sometimes towards you, my baby girl. I struggled like this for some time.

What I didn't understand at the time was that I had failed to grasp Ayurvedic teachings of addressing the root cause. I was focused narrowly on symptomology the way allopathic medicine often does. I assumed that indigestion could only be treated with what I am eating. It wasn't until I was able to talk about my fears surrounding life as a mother that we genuinely had a breakthrough. What did becoming a mom mean for me as an individual, and whether or not I was still going to be me and have my hopes and dreams that were solely my own?

In our coaching and bodywork sessions, I became aware of what I was holding in my body. The tension in my shoulders came from the harboring of pain from my relationship with my mother, who I knew loved me deeply, but had also recently hurt me deeply. Viji helped me realize this hurt bore out of my mom's struggles and wasn't really about me. The same way I wondered whether I would be able to separate myself from my child, I had now come to realize my mother, too, had her struggles. These sometimes manifested in our relationship. I, as her child, needed to separate her struggles from our relationship. This realization allowed me to separate my concerns and fears around motherhood and birth from my relationship with my child. This freedom, too, permeated into all other aspects of my life – not only did my digestion improve significantly, but I felt lighter and happier. And feeling well meant I took good care of my body; I had energy and excitement and a newfound appreciation for everyone and everything in my life, especially this special time I had with my baby growing inside me.

The impact of honoring the mind-body connection could not be overstated and led to the most incredible birth experience that I could not have even imagined. Ayurveda gave me the tools, Viji showed me the way, you gave me the motivation, and I took the steps.

For me, the journey into Ayurveda was a journey to self-connection, self-love, self-growth, self-healing, and ultimately self-empowerment. It helped me bridge the gap of heart, mind, and body that I wasn't even aware had become disconnected. I hope you know how valuable this connection is and come to learn of the power you possess.

Wherever you are in your divine journey, I hope you know that you are not defined by a singular moment in time. Life is a continual process of growth. You are the summation of thousands of years of experience, reflection, and growth. With you, you carry the teachings and knowledge of all of your ancestors before you. Take from it what you will and add to it as you please. Each day brings a new opportunity to redefine yourself as you continue on your journey.

Like Elaine, most of my clients have the birth of their dreams and desires, and in turn, have the experience of rebirthing themselves. Many of my clients heal generational trauma and begin to feel profound confidence in themselves and their bodies. Changes they have made directly impact these women's lives and their relationships with their partners and, most importantly, their babies.

CHAPTER TWO

Redefining Birth: From Moment to Journey

*"When you change the way you view birth,
the way you birth will change."*

- Marie F. Mongan

Birth is not a single moment in time as you are continually giving birth to yourself every day. You have the opportunity and ability to change and create within yourself with every sunrise. And as you work on and connect further with yourself, you are also preparing your body to give birth to your child. When you see birth as a journey and something that you experience every day, you open up the possibility to support it from different perspectives to be the best it can be!

As you embark on the journey of parenthood, examine how you view, understand, and approach birth. Throughout my years of supporting women, I have seen most people haphazardly arrive at pregnancy. For some, it is an unexpected, oops! For others, they have felt the pressure from family or society and decide to have kids because they 'should.' It's a natural 'next step,' and there is a push to continue the legacy of their forefathers and foremothers. Some women try very hard to get pregnant for years and struggle to get there. The unifying outlook for most is that they see it as a one-day event to happen. Most do not know or think about the details between conception and birth and certainly not postpartum. The day after the baby arrives, parents often find themselves unprepared for what follows.

Why is this? The modern cultural outlook on birth views it as a one-day event. We don't even have the cultural infrastructure to support mothers in the delicate postpartum. Arguably more important than a wedding, a baby's birth does not get the same amount of attention, time, energy, investment, or forethought. We decide to either prepare for our pregnancies by scouring the endless abyss of information and 'experts' via the internet or leave things to chance by showing up and hoping for the best. However, like a wedding, sometimes we choose to outsource to experts, like an event planner, who can help make the process easier or smoother. In childbirth, it would be a doula, midwife, or me, a coach, healer, and Ayurvedic practitioner. But is it worth the investment and effort? Does it help? Does it empower us to make better decisions and be the parents we want to be? How do we ensure the best circumstances for our birth and for the new life to be born? What type of experience are we creating for the baby? Are we leaving things to chance?

I can help you answer all of these questions. And for such a milestone for you, your partners, and your baby, leave as little to chance as possible.

Birth is and should be considered the most important event of one's lifetime. In so doing, it is paramount that we see birth for what it is. It is the journey of a lifetime - for you and the being you create. The journey is the sum of all of the events that led us to the moment and everything that follows. Every moment is an opportunity to recognize the continuation of birth and rebirth. In its entirety, birth is truly a journey, a divine one.

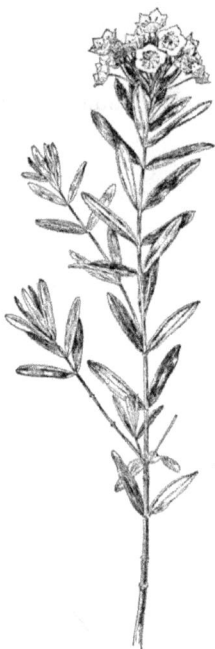

CHAPTER THREE

The Garden Within

"A garden requires patient labor and attention. Plants do not grow merely to satisfy ambitions or to fulfill good intentions. They thrive because someone expended effort on them."

- Liberty Hyde Bailey

Understanding birth as a journey, we should view our bodies as a garden that requires tending. Taking care of it is a daily activity. To manage it properly, you must know what it needs to thrive. You can use this knowledge to provide the best circumstances for a healthy body, mind, and spirit - a thriving garden!

When you plant seeds in the garden, some are no larger than a speck of dirt. But weeks later, with the right care, you will see it grow into a beautiful plant. Can you imagine that everything that would define this plant was all in that little speck? It is magical how these tiny seeds eventually form the stem, the leaves, the flower, and the fruit. A plant that would become strong and resilient came from a fragile speck of a seed. It's an incredible process of growth and transformation. Later, as you tend to it, you will notice all the factors that go into keeping the plant alive. The environment surrounding it, the elements of nature, and the nutrients to nourish it all play a role in its survival.

You have the role of being the caretaker of your inner garden. Do you pay attention to where you are planted? What do you feed yourself to grow and thrive? What environmental factors out of your control are affecting you? Like a plant, do you know which parts are ok to ignore, and which parts are necessary for your future survival and what is harmful?

And what about your baby? By the time you are 20 weeks pregnant, your baby's garden is already being formed. A baby girl has the seeds for her garden as follicles within her reproductive system! The connection of the body to future generations is mind-blowing.

Remember that the master gardener plans her garden, understands its needs, and recognizes nature's connection to grow and live in synergy with it. Within you is the seed of your baby. You will nurture it, and you will tend to it, birth it, and care for it. Learning how to take care of your garden will help you care for the beautiful creation you birth and set your baby up for generations to come.

CHAPTER FOUR

Tending the Garden using Ayurveda

*"The glory of gardening: hands in the dirt, head in the sun,
heart with nature. To nurture a garden is to feed
not just on the body, but the soul."*

-Alfred Austin

I invite you to pause and look at every endeavor you have ever undertaken in the past. Very few things happen in isolation, and most situations are affected by the circumstances leading up to and surrounding it. Both life and birth are the cumulative manifestations of the results of events, emotions, and circumstances that we (and our ancestors) have ever experienced. Life is a continuous and impactful journey; you live today, knowing it will impact tomorrow. We all are affected by our parents' journey. And our children are influenced by ours.

Preparing Ground

If you ever experienced starting a garden for the first time, you know that tons of books, blogs, and websites will painstakingly help you consider every aspect of building it! The decisions you make are numerous and influence such things as the types of plants you can grow, how many you can grow, and how they grow. Preparing ground for your garden is critical, and forethought goes a long way to success.

When planning for your baby and your birth, it is crucial to understand your body or the physical foundation of your garden. Society teaches us that we are stuck with the body we have. To a large extent, that is true, but we do have the power to influence the body and its environment. We can also influence the bodies that we create for our children. We are continuously developing and affecting our bodies; our ovum's genetic and physiological makeup changes. And through our thoughts, body, and spirit, you can consciously create the mind and body of your baby.

Ayurveda's ancient medical science provides the holistic outlook and roadmap for you first to understand the ground you are working with and then give it the best chance of supporting fertility and nurturing life both within and outside your body.

Tending

The environment around us, the macrocosm, gives us great insight into our health, body, and mind. It is easy to understand our inner world when we look at the outer one. When tending to a garden, you will know first-hand the amount of care and energy that goes into its maintenance. Tending requires you to bring a new level of awareness to your body. A plant needs good soil with nutrients, water, sunlight, and protection. These are the basics. And, like your own body, there are many more subtle factors to consider when you get beyond these basics.

Have you ever felt that your body is failing you? I've heard this from many women, and I urge them not to give up. It is not always the case that our body is not working. It is more accurate to know that your body just may not be functioning at its optimum, and you may not be doing what it needs to thrive. Often, people don't know and understand what their body requires. Most people follow what the crowd does, what comes up in a Google search, or what worked for their friend. Remember, we are all unique individuals, and no two people are alike. Even no two headaches are the same as so many factors can cause them. There are at least 17 classifications for headaches for a reason! And that being true, no two people will have the same remedy work the same as someone else.

Like your garden, where at first, you may be a little carefree in your initial inspection, you will start to be more observant. This newfound awareness is critical when you tend to the inner garden of your mind, body, and spirit in supporting your birth journey. It will allow you to identify what influences disturb you or create is available to provide support.

Being on the Journey and Ayurveda

When you desire to trust in and take care of your body without drugs, the tools from Ayurveda allow us to incorporate the natural wisdom available to us. We can superimpose and implement our understanding of the birth journey to the science's natural healing modalities.

In expanding our understanding of birth, we will no longer separate it from the emotional, physical, and spiritual influences that affect us. We begin to acknowledge and recognize what came before and see how our current and future actions can impact the birth trajectory and life journey. We, as humans, have the unique paradigm of embodying the garden and being our own gardener. The science of Ayurveda allows us to embrace this principle and prepare our body, mind, and spirit for the birth of our dreams. It begins with the lineage of our ancestors and continues into our progeny. When you prepare for your birth journey, remember that it is about your entire being, your existence's wholeness and the entirety of the journey—everything before you and everything after you is connected. Ayurveda connects existence, science, the mind, and spirit to allow you to influence your journey.

Preparation and nurturing yourself even before pregnancy have a significant influence over birth. Birth is not just about the baby; it is also about the mother, the entire family unit, and future generations. Many people carry generational trauma of which they are not aware of and unknowingly pass emotional, mental, and physical baggage onto their children, affecting them for the rest of their lives. Addressing these through the inner work of Ayurveda and creating health within oneself allows us to create health for future generations.

CHAPTER FIVE

Introduction to Ayurveda

"When diet is wrong, medicine is of no use.
When diet is correct, medicine is of no need."

-*Ayurvedic Proverb*

Ayurvedic medicine acknowledges and supports every part of a person's existence. It is the most elegant science to support your journey of birth. Like any medical system, the field of Ayurveda is extensive and takes a lifetime to master and understand. However, a brief introduction to the science is essential in understanding how Ayurveda's foundations can effectively support your birth journey.

Ayurvedic Medicine is a healing medical science based on the philosophy of balance in all body systems. It utilizes diet, natural herbal medicine, lifestyle treatments, and therapies, including yoga and meditation, to create true health. In Ayurvedic practice, a holistic understanding of a person is the foundation. Recommendations focus on looking at the root cause of one's illness or discomfort and not masking or temporarily addressing symptoms alone. Ayurveda not only treats a person's physical complaints, but it also addresses lifestyle practices to help maintain or improve physical, mental, and emotional health.

Like the garden, the union of seeds and the plant's nature are all influenced by the quality and nature of the process's supportive elements. Consider both the egg and sperm as the precious seeds, the mother's uterus the soil, the nourishment for the baby as the water, and perhaps most important and rarely considered, the time for conception or sowing.

Ayurveda's basics understand three functional forces or doshas in the body known as kapha, pitta, and vata. These are forces made of the primordial elements (air, fire, earth, water, ether) and are involved in creating, sustaining, and degrading the body. Doshas are present in the potential form before conception in both the egg and sperm that made you. These gametes contained a specific combination of the doshas, influenced by your parents' mental, physical, and spiritual health at the time of conception. This combination of doshas gave rise to your constitution.

The doshas then manifest in physical form when a baby is born and is responsible for the body's structural features and mental, emotional, and physiological functioning. Very much like one thinks of body types (meso, endo, ecto-morph), each person will usually have a predominance of one or two doshas that govern the functioning of their body and mind. This proportional makeup is known as your prakriti in Sanskrit or your constitution. Because they are the life energies behind all functioning in the body, one's constitution determines their emotional, physical, and functional attributes.

Knowing and understanding your constitution provides insight into the normal structure and functioning of your body and mind. It is your blueprint, and when you live life respecting and honoring and understanding that blueprint, you don't do things that will cause harm. From the moment we start interacting with the world, we are affected by it. When we do things that support our constitution and align with our constitution, we continue and support health. When we do something or experience things that could aggravate our constitution or cause imbalance, this is called vikruti. While prakriti does not change, vikruti can. Living per and supporting our prakriti helps us not to have ill health and create a vikruti.

In the context of Women's reproductive health, Ayurveda has a beautiful and straightforward way of addressing the complexity of interconnected networks in the body. In a pregnant mom, depending on her constitution (prakriti) and imbalance (vikruti), she is more likely to have certain complications during pregnancy, have her pregnancy go a certain way, and have specific postpartum issues. Through Ayurveda, you can identify any problems in advance, which gives you the ability to address these issues before they even arise! By understanding your mind, body, and spirit, you can better understand your constitution, which is the key to unlocking the roadmap to a magnificent birth and rebirth journey.

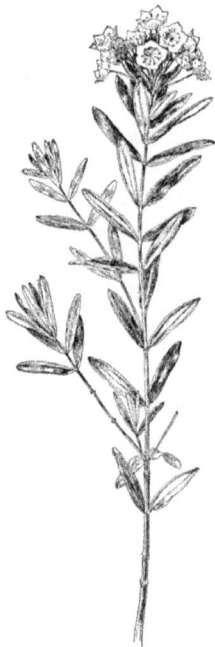

CHAPTER SIX

What is your Constitution?

"Knowing yourself is the beginning of all wisdom."

-Aristotle

Ayurveda considers health very individualistic, varying with each person's constitution (prakriti) and surrounding influences. One's body constitution is classified based on the predominance of one or more of the three doshas, kapha, pitta, and vata. The dominant dosha in an individual and nature, at the time, determines the health care provided to the individual.

The idea of your constitution is to understand what type of plant you are and identify the optimum conditions for your garden. When you know what factors aggravate or help you, you can be empowered to make the choices aligned with those.

Although not extensive, utilize this quick questionnaire to survey yourself and determine the predominant forces governing your mind, body, and spirit. In the next chapter, this information will help you to support your body with best practices and will help you to minimize common complaints during and after pregnancy. It is always best to understand and make these choices with a trained Ayurvedic Doctor and practitioner as your partner and guide.

If the following tool is challenging, here's another quick and general way to see where your energies tend to lie:

- A kapha predominant person tends to be on the cooler side but has a solid and heavy frame. Lovely curvy women are kapha, and they tend to gain weight easily. They are slow, calm, deliberate, and can even be stubborn. Kapha people are stable and don't change based on influence quickly.

- A predominant pitta person tends to be the hot type! You have a medium body frame and tend to heated things like inflammation, acne, rashes, looser stools, acidity, anger, and generally have a Type A personality.

- A vata predominant person tends to be cold and has a thin and lean body frame. You tend to have cold hands and feet and deal with insomnia, anxiety, worry, spaciness, constipation, or are easily pushed in any direction.

Please mark which one(s) from each category describes you the best. With time or due to changes one implements, one could see changes in their body. To identify your constitution, look at long term tendencies and behavior and not current disturbances.

Total up the attributes that describe you from each column. The first column describes more vata tendencies, the second pitta, and the third kapha.

Attributes	Vata	Pitta	Kapha
Body Frame	Thin, lanky, slim with lean muscles	Medium, symmetrical with good muscle development	Stocky, round, broad, or large
Weight	Lose easily	Constant weight	Gain easily
Hips	Slender, thin	Medium	Wide, Heavy
Schedule	Irregular schedule/eating times	Long workday	Good at keeping a routine
Sleep	Light sleeper	Sleep well, average length	Deep, long, trouble waking
Appetite	Irregular/small	Strong hunger	Steady, moderate

Thirst	Irregular	Strong and frequently	Rarely Thirsty
Digestion	Gas, irregular	Steady, strong	Slow, heavy
Skin	Thin	Warm and rosy	Thick, cool
Hair	Dry, dark, frizzy	Fine, straight, light, reddish	Thick, wavy
Eyes	Sunken, small, active, dark	Sharp, gray, green, light brown	Large, calm, loving
Lips	Thin	Bright red lips,	Large, smooth
Speech	Talks quickly	Sharp language	Slow speech
Emotions	Anxiety, fear, uncertainty	Anger, irritable, ambitious, analytical	Calm, attached, stagnant
Mood	Mood changes quickly	Intense emotions	Steady emotions
Personality	Creative, imaginative	Intelligent, efficient, perfectionist	Caring, calm, patient
Response to Conflict	Restlessness	Angry, irritable	Depressed, lazy

Social	Make and change friends often	Friends are work-related, change with job	Friendships are long-lasting, sincere
Stamina	Short bursts of energy	Medium	Steady, high
Climate	Avoids cold	Avoids heat	Avoids humidity
Activity	Hyperactive, quick	Moderate pace, goal-oriented	Slow, steady
Your Totals:			

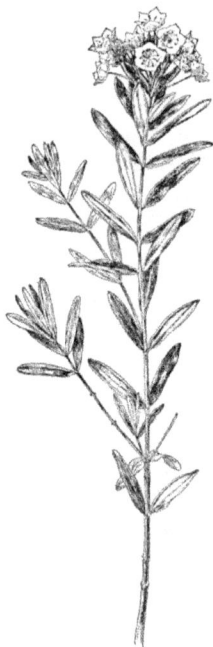

CHAPTER SEVEN

How your Constitution can
Influence your Pregnancy

"We have to know our place in the ecosystem of which we are a part, and this means living 'consciously': being aware of nature and how it affects us and how we, in turn, affect nature."

-Sebastian Pole

Pregnancy is a time of significant change in a woman's body. The types of symptoms or disturbances you experience indicate the dosha at play and cause these symptoms. Remember, doshas are the predominant forces in the body that govern structure, function, and emotions. Thus, depending on your dominant doshas and the lifestyle practices you have, the way your body responds to pregnancy will be different. Having this knowledge can empower you to make choices that support you. You can work with an Ayurvedic Practitioner to address symptoms that arise to connect them back to food, lifestyle, events, climate, and other factors. In my practice, women have overcome cysts, endometriosis, hypothyroidism, gestational diabetes, cholestasis, and more! These successes were all based on supporting the energetic factors that were out of balance. To this, you will need the help of a skilled practitioner to guide you.

Now that you have a sense of your predominant dosha or doshas, let's see how these can play out in pregnancy. In the tables that follow, you can see how a dosha predominance in your constitution can manifest physically.

Kapha Mama

Physical Nature	• Broad, heavy, evenly framed • Thick and oily hair, skin, nails • Easy to gain weight, hard to lose
Personality	• Slow, deliberate speech • Stable, calm, attached, stubborn • Careful but easy-going about making decisions • Prefers others to start projects; likes working on them
Appetite	• Likes to eat • Can go without eating without discomfort

Elimination	• Well-formed, slow and easy stools • ~ 1 bowel movement per day without straining
Typical Issues Faced During Pregnancy	• Heaviness • Breathlessness • Greater weight gain • Water retention • Extra growths • Yeast issues • Dullness in the mind • Lethargy • Gestational Diabetes
Labor Pattern	• Not complicated • Can have water retention • Going past the due date
Activities That Will Support	• Calming meditation • Breathing exercises • Massage with nurturing oils, especially during labor • Mental preparedness exercises such as hypnosis • Moderate walking, swimming, yoga
Food Guidelines	• Dry, toasted bread, but try to avoid simple carbohydrates • Milk should be taken warm with a small amount of ginger and cardamom milk • Most astringent fruits are good. Minimize sweet and sour fruit. • Raw vegetables during the summer; cooked at other times • Foods should be well spiced.

Pitta Mama

Physical Nature	• Medium and proportionate • Fine, oily hair • Penetrating eyes; sensitive to light • Pink, well-formed nails • Easy to gain, easy to lose
Personality	• Decisive and articulate speech • Can be aggressive, irritable • Easy to make decisions • Likes to start and finish projects
Appetite	• Good or intense appetite • Can get irritable or angry if missed a meal • Excessive thirst
Elimination	• Looser Stools
Typical Issues Faced During Pregnancy	• Increased body heat/sweating • Acidity or acid reflux or heartburn • Indigestion • Inflammation • Infections • Cholestasis • Pre-eclampsia • Trouble falling asleep • Anger and irritability • Bleeding Issues
Labor Pattern	• Could go faster than average • Blood pressure spikes • Increased bleeding

Activities That Will Support	• Calming meditation • Breathing exercises • Massage with nurturing oils, especially during labor • Mental preparedness exercises such as hypnosis • Moderate walking, swimming, yoga
Food Guidelines	• Grains should be cooked • Bread should not be yeasted • Milk should be taken warm with a small amount of ginger and cardamom • Sweeter fruits are best. Avoid sour fruits. • Cooked, sweet, and bitter vegetables are best; avoid pungent vegetables • Legumes that have been soaked for a long time and spiced • Lightly roasted and only very slightly salted nuts best • Healthy Oils • Avoid spicy and acidic foods • Warm or room temperature beverages

Vata Mama

Physical Nature	<ul><li>Lean and small frame</li><li>Dry hair, skin, nails</li><li>Hard to gain weight, easy to lose</li></ul>
Personality	<ul><li>Can be talkative and speak fast</li><li>Tend to worry or be more overwhelmed</li><li>Have difficulty making decisions</li><li>Likes to start projects but finds it difficult to finish</li></ul>
Appetite	<ul><li>Variable appetite</li><li>Can get lightheaded, anxious, or cranky if missed a meal</li></ul>
Elimination	<ul><li>Dry, harder stools and tend towards constipation</li><li>Experience gas, bloating</li></ul>
Typical Issues Faced During Pregnancy	<ul><li>Nausea and hyperemesis</li><li>Anemia</li><li>Anxiety, Worry, Overwhelm</li><li>Increased darker regions of the body</li><li>Vaginal dryness</li><li>Increased pain, especially in joints and bones</li><li>May feel exhausted/low energy</li><li>Become absent-minded</li><li>Poor circulation</li></ul>
Labor Pattern	<ul><li>Experience more pain</li><li>Smaller pelvis</li><li>Longer labors</li><li>Uncoordinated contractions</li><li>Difficulty in baby's descent</li></ul>

Activities That Will Support	<ul><li>Calming meditation</li><li>Breathing exercises</li><li>Massage with nurturing oils, especially during labor</li><li>Mental preparedness exercises such as hypnosis</li><li>Moderate walking, swimming, yoga</li><li>Lots of rest, going to bed early</li><li>Regular daily routine</li><li>Food/drinks/body should be warm</li><li>Cooked and slightly oily food</li><li>Slower/relaxing activities</li><li>Yoga, meditation, quiet time</li></ul>
Food Guidelines	<ul><li>Grains should be cooked</li><li>Bread should not be yeasted</li><li>Milk should be taken warm with a small amount of ginger and cardamom</li><li>Sweeter fruits are best</li><li>Cooked vegetables</li><li>Legumes that have been soaked for a long time</li><li>Lightly roasted nuts best</li><li>Healthy Oils</li><li>Warm or room temperature beverages</li></ul>

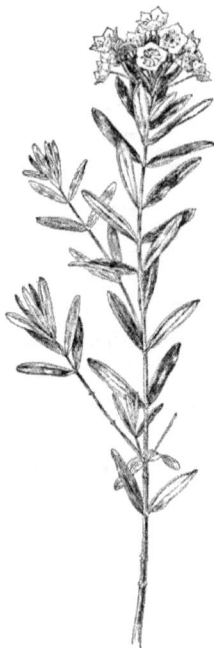

CHAPTER EIGHT

Creating the Foundation of Your Garden:
Ayurvedic Practices to Support Your Birth
Journey

You can't build a great building on a weak foundation.
You must have a solid foundation
if you're going to have a strong superstructure.

-Gordon B. Hinckley

You can do simple and powerful techniques every day to create a healthy environment in your body. In all stages of one's birth journey, the proper functioning of the doshas is essential. Whether you would like to get pregnant, keep your baby thriving, or support the delivery and postpartum recovery process, each tip allows the body to come into energetic balance and function properly physiologically. It will help you birthing a healthy baby and create health and healing for your own body.

Here are some guidelines to help you implement these practices. Think of this as the foundational factors to set up your garden.

It is vital to establish a routine, and doing these practices every day consistently will help create a positive and supportive environment. However, the stress of not doing them or missing a day is counterproductive. Start by implementing one practice at a time so that it does not feel overwhelming. Have each tip develop into a habit and then add one more at a time.

Remember, there is no one size fits all, and each plant has its different needs. This book allows you to understand and lay the foundation for working deeper with a practitioner for your individual needs. Therefore, the plan is never finite and can evolve with time. When external factors such as climate, stress, and food changes impact your body, modifications will be needed to bring you back on track. No matter what, these foundational tips will support you in creating mental peace and physical stability.

PRACTICE 1: CREATE A ROUTINE

As simple as it may sound, very few people have a routine. However, bringing structure to your daily activities allows all body functions to be regulated. It helps to create a habit that can provide stability to your mind as well as the body. Whenever we build healthy habits, we train our bodies and mind. It's tough to summon the body to perform upon request. Allowing yourself to develop strengths over time consistently is the best way to be ready for anything that comes your way.

Daily practice allows these healthy habits to become a part of you, and they will strongly support you in times of duress. The prenatal period is critical, and you can significantly influence both your baby and your body. During this time, you build the baby's body, mind, and spirit, so it is essential to support yourself and your baby through healthy practices.

A daily prenatal routine will help you balance your body's energies, calm your mind, connect to your baby, check-in with yourself, regulate digestion, and increase circulation. These practices may appear simple, but they will contribute to you having a smoother pregnancy as well as smoother labor and delivery. When a woman gets pregnant, there are many body changes. Vata and pitta doshas increase significantly due to the speed at which cell division and biological miracles are creating the baby! The very nature of having routine addresses and balances vata in the body.

Don't give yourself a hard time if you miss some of the components or miss the routine altogether. Your goal is to try and get back on track to incorporate lasting lifestyle changes. If you miss something one day, tomorrow is a NEW day! It is not about perfection but consistency and incorporating these healing measures to increase overall health in mind, body, and spirit.

Once you establish a routine, you will notice how you may feel different at certain times of the day. Ayurveda understands that our body and its rhythms align with the times of the day. Specific times of the day are associated with particular doshas and their energies and specific organs in the body. Doshas affect the entirety of our being, including our emotions and their fluctuations throughout the day. Paying attention can help you understand what is happening in your body on a deeper level. The body's energetic clock allows you to know how to support yourself at different times of the day. Discuss further with an Ayurvedic Doctor for more details.

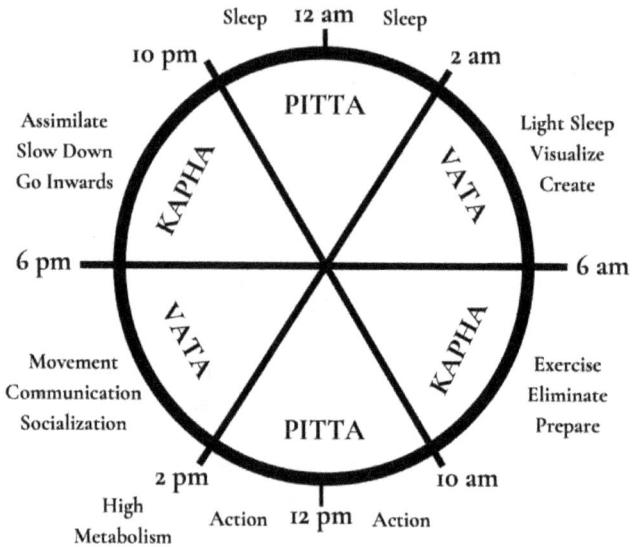

A few guidelines for creating a daily routine:

1. Wake up at the same time every day.
2. Set a daily intention.
3. Do not hold in urges (sneezing, coughing, during, passing, gas).
4. Spend time in nature.
5. Go to bed at the same time every day.
6. Promote healthy sleep with a bedtime ritual.

PRACTICE 2: OIL PULL

The practice of oil pulling is an ancient Ayurvedic practice used to eliminate waste from the body without destroying one's healthy microflora. Based on the principle that like dissolves like, oil pulling dissolves toxins and plaque in the mouth. Did you know that the Charaka Samhita, an ancient Ayurvedic text, expounds that this practice cures 30 systemic diseases of the body? Some of these include headaches and migraines, diabetes, and asthma! Traditional Indian households have used the technique for foul mouth odor, bleeding gums, throat dryness, cracked lips, and strengthening the teeth, gums, and jaw. My clients have said that oil pulling improved their sense of taste and even teeth color!

I recommend this practice because when we bathe the mouth in oil, we also influence the tongue. Like in traditional Chinese medicine, the tongue is believed to be connected to every organ in the body. This practice allows you to cleanse, purify, and support it.

In Ayurveda, sesame oil is typically used and has been well studied for safety and efficacy. You can also do oil pulling with coconut oil, which is naturally antibacterial and has a milder taste. Some prefer to add a drop or two of essential oils like peppermint.

To begin, swish organic unrefined sesame oil in your mouth for 5 to 15 minutes, moving the oil around your teeth and side to side. The oil may foam up initially. You can spit some out if you start to feel uncomfortable. It's a practice that requires time to become familiar. After the swishing is complete, spit out the oil in the trash. Avoid spitting the oil into the sink or toilet, as this may clog your pipes. Rinse your mouth well with water before eating or drinking anything.

PRACTICE 3: SCRAPE YOUR TONGUE

The tongue can tell you a lot about your body. In traditional Indian and Chinese medicine, the tongue represents the body. Examining it provides a lens into what is going on inside. When you wake up in the morning, do you notice a thin or thick film on your tongue? Does it change color from one day to another? According to Ayurveda, this coating reveals your digestive health. Digestive toxins or ama, in Sanskrit, are the result of undigested and unprocessed foods. These manifest on the tongue as a coating and gives you insight into your health.

Ama means that which harms or weakens. When ama overflows from the digestive system, it enters and coats the body's cells and can interfere with tissue functioning. Therefore, the simple process of scraping your tongue can help remove these toxins. Gently scraping the tongue stimulates and improves your internal organs' health by eliminating bacteria, improving oral hygiene, freshening breath, and cleansing the taste buds.

For reference, a white coating relates to a kapha related digestive issue, yellow indicating pitta disorders, and gray relating to problems with vata. The thickness of the layer indicates the relative strength of your digestive capabilities. The thinner the coating, the better your digestion.

Beyond just the coating, one can also utilize the tongue to understand different disorders of the body. A discoloration or sensitivity in particular areas indicates a disruption in the organ corresponding to that area. On the next page, you can see in the picture of the tongue that the front one-third of the tongue relates to the lungs, heart, chest, and neck. The central third of the tongue refers to the liver, spleen, stomach, and pancreas and the rear one-third area of the tongue relates to the lower abdominal organs, such as the small intestine and colon. If a coating covers this back part of the tongue, that is ama or toxins in the colon, indicating low colon energy.

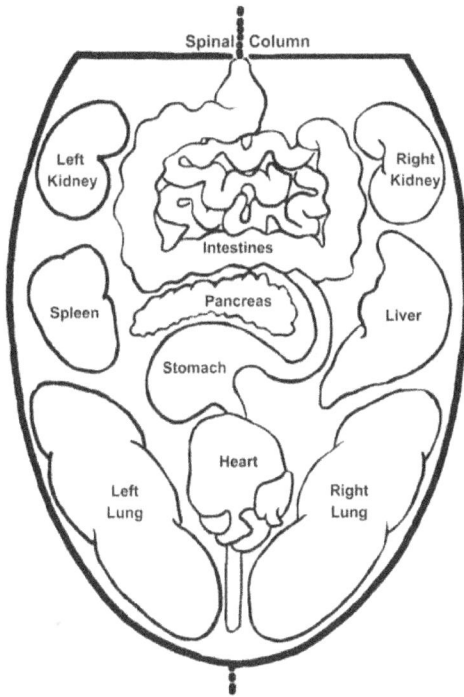

Spinal Column

Left Kidney

Right Kidney

Intestines

Spleen

Pancreas

Liver

Stomach

Heart

Left Lung

Right Lung

How to Scrape Your Tongue:

Start by holding the tongue scraper by both ends. Extend your tongue out and place the tongue scraper as far back as you feel comfortable. Gently bring the scraper down to the tip. Rinse the scraper with water and then repeat. Don't press too hard or do too many repetitions to avoid damaging your tongue. It's ideal to do this first thing in the morning—on an empty stomach and before your brush your teeth.

PRACTICE 4: SELF MASSAGE

Abhyanga or Ayurvedic hot oil massage, although perhaps the most famous Ayurvedic treatment, is often overlooked because of its simplicity. This practice has many benefits and is not about pampering or overindulgence! It is about restoring and supporting the health of your body and baby.

The gentle repetition and warmth of your massage strokes help move waste out of the cells and through the channels for elimination, and it supports all systems to work better. It also takes a mother deeper into her mind-body connection, into those places which we so easily ignore in our outer responsibility and often not well understood, inner, invisible work.

Remember that every practice in Ayurveda focuses on the individual and understands what one needs to support their body. The skin is the largest organ, and it is easy to affect our body through the skin. On the most foundational level, daily body massage with appropriate oils for your body constitution is an important practice that brings in the quality of self-love and self-acceptance. Over time, it allows you to become deeply connected with yourself and your baby. It helps to calm both the mind and body and will enable the body to heal even by any dis-ease caused by mental disturbances and chatter.

On a physiological level, self-massage increases circulation, aids in digestion, reduces body pain, prevents early aging and stress, and lubricates the joints to alleviate degenerative issues such as rheumatoid arthritis. Self-massage contributes to balancing the three doshas in the body and correcting any deviation from normal that has arisen. Each massage stroke addresses marma or acupressure points connected with your body's organs and organ function. With the appropriate supportive oils, you can help to balance the entire functioning of the body.

Details on How to do Self Massage:

Begin by preparing and make sure that you have all the items you need. You will need an old sheet or towel that you can sit on while doing the massage. Make sure it covers the area that you are sitting on and a little bit more. You can also do this self-massage in the shower.

Choosing the best oil is based on your constitution (whether greater in kapha, pitta, or vata) and current complaints. You can also consult an Ayurvedic Doctor for more specific oils for you. Sesame oil is ideal for all doshas. It can penetrate deeply and nourish all the tissues. It also supports the process of fetal expulsion during delivery and the time of transition in the postpartum. Alternative choices for each dosha are listed below.

Dosha	Additional Oil Recommendations
Kapha	Mustard Oil or kapha massage oil to decrease heaviness
Pitta	Coconut Oil or pitta massage oil to decrease heat
Vata	Almond oil or vata massage oil to decrease dryness, cold

*You can find dosha specific massage oils at Banyan Botanicals and other Ayurvedic Suppliers

First, transfer the oil to a glass bottle. Do not heat plastic containers. Warm the oil by placing the bottle in hot water or use your hands and rub them together actively.

To begin, pour a tablespoon of warm oil on your scalp. Using the flat part of your palm, not the fingertips, massage the oil into the scalp. Then, with circular strokes, cover the entire area of your scalp, similar to if you were shampooing your hair. Add more oil if needed. If you do not want to soak your hair with oil, it is ok to skip the head.

Move to your face and ears...
Massaging more gently, stroke across the forehead, slowly circle the temples, and then move to the backs of the ears. Follow the jaw and circle the cheeks—stroke across the upper lip and chin.

Apply a small amount of warm oil to your entire body.

Give attention to each part, noticing how you feel and if there is any tension or pain. Just observe and continue. The general rule of thumb is that you utilize circular motions on all joints and long strokes on all the limbs. Make sure not to miss any part as the body is our storage receptacle. We store physical issues and emotions in our bodies, and this daily practice will allow you to check-in and release anything you no longer need to hold.

Neck...
We carry much tension in our neck and shoulders. Massage back and forth and up and down the front and back of your neck. Circular strokes can also be helpful. Being mindful, please apply more or less pressure where you need it.

Arms and Hands...
Remember to use circular motions and the shoulders and elbow joints and long, back and forth strokes on the muscles. Massage the front and back of your hands, including the palm, and gently pull each finger, paying attention to the joints.

Chest and Abdomen...
Apply oil to the chest and abdomen with gentle sweeping strokes. Make sure to get the breasts and the axillary or armpit region as well. Use soft, circular motions on the belly in a clockwise direction to support bowel movement.

Back and Sides...
These areas may be hard to reach but apply oil to both the sides and the back without much strain. You may request help to reach your spine and other areas if needed.

Legs...
Remember, all joints, including the hip, are addressed through circles. Follow the hips with long strokes on the thigh. Stroke the sides, the front, and the back. Circular motion on the knees, long stroke down the legs, circles on the ankle bone, and gentle strokes up and down the leg and each toe!

Sit and allow the oil to soak in, and be with yourself. When you are ready, you can bathe or shower with warm water.

PRACTICE 5: DIGESTIVE TEA

The digestive system is the lens into your body and how it is functioning. Ayurveda believes all diseases begin in the digestive system. It may be hard to understand, but both a headache and Parkinson's' disease all start from an imbalance in the digestive system. When left unchecked and allowed to progress over time, it can affect the body's various organ systems. The digestive fire (or jataragni) is critical for the functioning of your body.

Your digestive fire should be able to properly and adequately break down the foods that you eat. Often, when we don't feel hungry or don't digest our food properly, this results from improper or imbalanced functioning of jataragni. Warm, digestive tea will be helpful to kindle the digestive fire. Start by boiling some coriander, cumin, and fennel in some water and drinking it in the morning (warm to room temperature). Pay attention to all aspects of your body and digestion, and even hunger levels.

Over time, you will notice that your tongue has less coating, you are hungry in the morning, and your stools may pass more regularly.

> ½ teaspoon cumin seeds
> ½ teaspoon coriander seeds
> ½ teaspoon fennel seeds
> 4–5 cups of water

Heat the water in a stainless-steel pot over high heat. Add the seeds. Allow the tea to boil for 5 to 10 minutes, depending on the preferred strength. Strain out the seeds, and drink hot or warm.

This tea is best made and taken fresh every day in the morning!

PRACTICE 6: BREATHING EXERCISES

Numerous medical studies have shown that breathing can help to regulate both the sympathetic and parasympathetic nervous systems. This regulation is essential to mitigate the stress response in the body. Stress can be attributed to causing most physical conditions and affects so many organ systems. Stress can cause anxiety and depression, thyroid issues, and fatigue. Breathing practices help to regulate the deranged movement of vata in both the mind and body. These practices will help to bring more awareness to your body and slow down the movement of thoughts. Cessation of thoughts in the mind helps the body to heal.

Pranayama:

Pranayama or breath control is an easily accessible practice that you can do anywhere and at any time. Many types of breathing practices are available. When you start your practice, begin by just sitting down in a comfortable position and observing your breath. Observe the inhales and exhales and do this for some time. This simple effort itself will allow you to bring mindfulness.

Next, you can try to do alternate nostril breathing, known as nadi shuddhi or cleansing breath. Inhaling through the left nostril triggers the rest/relaxation response (parasympathetic nervous system), and inhaling through the right stimulates the fight/flight response (sympathetic nervous system). Doing alternate nostril breathing can improve respiratory health, cardiovascular health, and reduce stress and anxiety by dampening the stress response. Taking the time to breathe reduces one's propensity to worry and ruminate when the breath becomes the focus.

Begin by inhaling to a count of 4 from one nostril, holding the breath for a count of 7, and then exhaling for eight from the other nostril. Alternate the inhale and exhale with each nostril.

Brhamari:

Brhamari is the breath of the bumblebee and is named from the sound made from the back of the throat when doing the practice. The practice balances the nervous system, stimulates the pineal and pituitary glands, and allows the breath to flow smoothly. Brhamari has been shown to relieve tension, anger and anxiety, hypertension, mitigates migraines, reduces blood pressure, and improves concentration and memory.

Begin by placing your thumbs on the cartilage between your cheek and ear. Using your thumb tip, close the opening of your ear by gently pressing the cartilage. Next, place your index & middle fingers gently over your eyes with the tips of your fingers between your inner eye and the bridge of your nose. Do not press down on your eyes. Then place the end of your ring finger gently above your nostrils and your pinky fingers just above your upper lip. Inhale through your nose and as you exhale, make a loud humming sound like a bee.

Sheetali:

Sheetali breath is also known as cooling breath. As the name implies, when the body and mind are heated, this practice can help cool you down. This type of breathing practice is suitable for any pitta disturbances one experiences.

Practice Sheetali by inhaling through a curled tongue and exhaling through the nose. During each exhalation through your nose, lightly touch the tip of the tongue to the roof of the mouth. Invite the cool tip of the tongue to send coolness toward the upper palate. Swallow now and then if the throat feels dry. Continue this cycle for one to five minutes—until you feel refreshed. If you are unable to curl your tongue, practice a variation known as Sheetkari pranayama. Do this by inhaling through the teeth, with the lips parted and the tongue floating just behind the teeth. Hold the breath for a few seconds and then exhale through your nose slowly.

PRACTICE 7: MEDITATION

Arguably, meditation has now become as mainstream as it was thousands of years ago. Researchers in various fields, including medicine, have concluded that meditation can be helpful in many conditions. These can be from sleep to blood pressure to fighting addiction. It is such an accessible practice and can be done anywhere at any time. You don't need a particular environment, props, or anything to do meditation.

So, what is meditation? Meditation is a process, better to be done regularly as a habit, to train the mind to focus, observe, and redirect your thoughts. It is a gathering of a combination of synergistic steps done together.

If you consider the season of pregnancy and birth, there are many positive benefits of incorporating meditation into your daily routine. First, it allows you to focus on and increase awareness of yourself and your baby. There is a deeper level of connection to yourself that activates when you let everything else go around you and focus inwards. It is common to have a greater inner perception of your thoughts and body functioning. Actively focusing allows one to be present and focus on the here and now. Not only does it improve your concentration ability, but it also allows you not to be a part of the mind's chatter about the past or the future. It allows you not to miss the present moment. Innately, this helps to reduce stress.

Once the inner awareness begins, it is possible to redirect our outlook and thoughts to create a positive vibration. Many of my clients have healed themselves of many physical ailments, such as cysts, high blood pressure, and other medical conditions, just using meditation. You will start to see your sleep patterns normalize and develop control over the physical body and sensations that you may experience. One sees their pain tolerance also increases.

PRACTICE 8: PRACTICE SURRENDER

Surrender is perhaps one of the most challenging things for us to do. Our culture values to go for what we want, exercise our voice, and get it! These are all excellent concepts and the adrenaline that rushes through us during monumental times in our life is there to help us push and move forward. However, there are circumstances in life, many as it turns out, that may not go exactly the way we envisioned it. It's true when they say, sometimes things don't turn out the way we want, but what happened was far better than we could have ever imagined.

Birth is one of those journeys that often teach us more than we ever thought would be possible. Your body and mind go through a process that may forever change you. You will experience the different stages of the process and show up differently to each one. The excitement preparation phase, the anxiety phase with anticipation, and then "when things start," I always advise my clients that it is best to be like the leaf in the wind. Allow your body to take you where it needs to go and surrender to its ultimate intelligence.

Many moms get frustrated with non-straightforward labors, disappointing expectations of a particular path, especially ones that don't go smooth or with a pause. The moment of surrender, true surrender, allows the ripe fruit to fall to the ground for us to enjoy.

Your release of expectations removes stress and attachment that allows ease in both the physical and emotional body to support the most uncomplicated birth you can have.

How does one practice surrender? Again, everything requires practice. Practicing every day in the small and subtle things that come up allows us to be ready to be less attached and let go.

PRACTICE 9: MOVEMENT

The physicality of birth is profoundly about the body and the flow of new life through it. Strength and flexibility are essential. We always hear that birth is like a marathon. Even this analogy demonstrates that endurance and adaptability are required. Like any marathon, one must train and prepare. Don't just show up and see how it goes!

Most people fear that movement is not suitable for pregnancy. Too many friends, family, and neighbors tend to comment to be careful. While it is essential to be mindful in early pregnancy, well-informed movement and physical activity help one to develop the endurance for the day of labor. Even the psychological part of the journey can be physically exhausting!

Your movement should be consistent and doesn't need to be intense. Begin by incorporating more exercise into your daily routine, just a little bit every day. You will slowly help build your stamina and strengthen muscles. From there, make sure to make walking a regular part of our routine. Towards the end of pregnancy, walking utilizes gravity to engage the baby, cervical thinning and loosening the joints.

Yoga should be a regular part of your daily routine. Yoga can develop strength, increase flexibility, and allows you to utilize your breath to connect to your body.

PRACTICE 10: PROCESS YOUR EMOTIONS

It sounds simple, but every experience we have impacts us. Whether positive or negative, we leave with impressions, either conscious or unconscious. These impressions can be both physical as well as emotional or psychological. Have you ever wondered when you are worried or nervous about something, why you may experience those "butterflies" in your stomach? This sensation is because there is a gut-brain connection, and we are connected physiologically to our emotions.

When we interact with the world, people and things inevitably affect us. Unfortunately, our experiences may not always be positive, and they may sometimes even be traumatic. Many of the events in our early years of life affect us profoundly. Over time, we develop coping mechanisms and behaviors to survive. However, some of the ways we've learned to manage life's difficult situations don't always serve us now.

It may be surprising to hear how many women overcame infertility, heal relationships with their partners, and have births that went smoothly due to identifying and processing emotionally challenging events from the past. It was difficult for them to see the connection or understand how harbored feelings affected their physical health. Over time and doing the inner work, they felt it was worth it when they saw a positive outcome.

When we experience difficult and troubling circumstances in life, we may internalize our emotions, which affects our physical health. It's essential to release the feelings stuck inside us to be better able to live joyful, present, and connected lives. The Emotional Processing Guide that follows will help you understand your feelings, undo self-destructive behaviors, and navigate how to move forward.

Begin by establishing a process of examining your feelings through journaling. Only you know best what is inside of you. Be your counselor, best friend, and sage. Learn to listen to your inner voice.

Although it may feel challenging to tap into your inner experiences, journaling will help you develop this relationship with yourself and access your feelings more easily. Start by journaling whenever you notice any unsettling feelings arise. If you come across a situation that makes you feel emotionally triggered or charged, find a space to spend a few minutes doing this practice. Use the following sequence to begin your processing.

1. What happened?
2. What am I feeling? (You are entitled to feel whatever you think, so write it down unfiltered and without judgment.)
3. What exactly made me feel this way? (It can be an action, word, or circumstance)
4. Towards whom am I feeling this way? (It might even be yourself)
5. What were this person's intentions?
6. Can I change or influence the situation in any way?
7. Where can I go from here? (Sit, turn inwards, and listen.)

It is often helpful to have a skilled practitioner who can help you process and connect the dots to your overall health. If you have a friend who knows you very well and whom you trust to be vulnerable, listen to their insight into what they may feel is an obstacle in your journey. However, even if done by yourself, processing allows you to understand why you feel a certain way (we don't always know), put things into perspective, and allows you to develop and hear your inner wisdom. Give it a try! It's simple and highly effective. It can change your life!

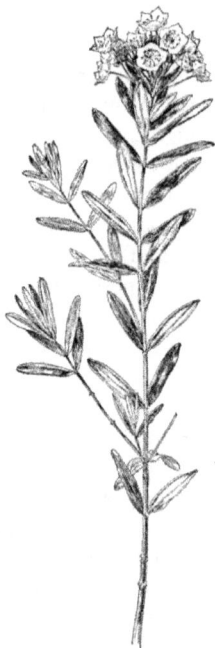

CHAPTER NINE

Closing Words

"You can't build a great building on a weak foundation.
You must have a solid foundation
if you're going to have a strong superstructure."

-Gordon B. Hinckley

Throughout our lives, we take part in creating an environment in our bodies. We have the canvas we are born with, and along with our choices and actions, we influence this environment. We can create good health by living according to and supporting our constitution, and aggravating our constitution through influences that affect our body, mind, and spirit results in ill-health. External stresses like work, personal issues of worry and disappointment, and consuming foods that are not supportive can result in physical problems in the body.

As we go through life, pay attention to your lifestyle and routines. Notice how they may affect how you feel. There will always be times where we do not have control. We may not be able to change external circumstances, but it is possible to incorporate healing measures to minimize these disturbances. During troubled times, it is easy to forget and abandon your self-care the most. Prioritize your mental as well as physical health as the primary goal. Simple practices can help to address the root causes.

You have the power to architect a thriving garden. When you tend to your inner garden of well-being, you can grow a healthy and resilient life. Like the plant that regrows even after you have plucked a leaf or trimmed it entirely, you are in a continual cycle of birth and rebirth every day. As the informed gardener, when you see your entire life as your birth journey, you can have the power to create health within continually. Your thriving garden will be a strong foundation to give birth and support your baby's health.

If you are interested in exploring your health further with Divine Journey, we happily serve women worldwide. Please visit us at
www.divinejourney.me